NAVIGATING NICO: A COLLECTION OF GIFTS FROM MY SON

Dana Bauer

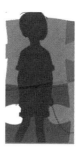

Cover design by: Justin Pasquinelli
Front cover photo by: Bethanie Weigel, Bethanie Photography
Back cover photo gy: Bethanie Weigel, Bethanie Photography
Courage in a Dog photo by: Courtney Ferraro
A Bow on the Top photo by Courney Ferraro
About the Author photo by: Bethanie Weigel, Bethanie Photography
ISBN: 978-0-578-80236-7
Library of Congress Control Number: TXu 2-218-449
Printed in the United States of America

To my inspriation, my gift, my son-I love you to the stars.

CONTENTS

FOREWORD

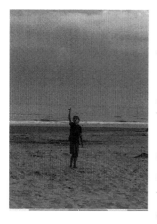

Gifts. Most of us unofficially define them as things that are special, objects that bring us great joy. Most of the time, they are given with love, from a place of pure intention. Take the picture on the front of this book and the one to the left.Pictures taken as dusk took over the Atlantic coast, at a small beach town in New Jersey. A family vacation took us to this touristy town full of noise, food, and fun. Nico had received a kite the day prior, a gift from his grandmother. Wanting to take it out for a test flight proved too challenging during the day, as beach goers made it so the sand was too crowded. We waited until dusk and trudged through the soft sand to the ocean's edge. We unwrapped the white string from the red handle, slowly, and before we knew it, the wind caught the multicolored diamond, taking it swiftly high into the sky, its colors brilliantly fanned in front of the grey clouds and pink sunset. Nico, smiled at the kite, with all of his face and soul, in a way only he can, his eyes sparkling much like the water was behind him. He was happy, this gift bringing him joy. He squealed in delight, time standing still. He was alone in his space, delighted, and at peace. This kite, this gift, spreading happiness, a sense of peace, and an almost whimsical sense of inspiration as it dipped and rose with the winds, without doing anything but being itself, doing what it was designed to do. Nothing more, nothing less. And it was spectacular. This story, of Nico flying his kite at dusk, right before we turned in for the night, inspired me to write this book. This book is a collection of stories, of gifts, given to me from my son. Each story is a celebration of Nico, of the fight that lies within, and the lessons that he has taught us, all from being nothing more than who he was meant to be, and from doing exactly what he was designed to do. Nothing more, nothing less. And he is, indeed, spectacular.

THE GREEN BICYCLE

Outside play, when one is a child, is a magical thing. The fresh air, the sunshine, the freedom. Something about playing outside spells out childhood in a way not many other activities can. Bike riding is especially popular in our neighborhood, which is equipped with many sidewalks and side streets on which very few cars travel. Many children in our subdivision enjoy carefree weekend days and weekday evenings riding down hills, biking to their friends' houses to see if they are free for a playdate, or racing other children around corners and through grass. Nico's brother had gotten a bike for his birthday and took to riding it quite easily. His brother had picked out a red and black bicycle, and before long, had shed the training wheels, riding around the neighborhood almost effortlessly in a matter of days. Watching his brother ride his new bike sparked an interest in Nico. He expressed that he, too, would like to have a bike, and so, on a rainy day in March, we took Nico to the store to pick out a bicycle of his own.

We pulled up to the store, placing our hoods on our heads to combat the rain, and I took Nico's hand as he stepped out of our van, a smile on his face. He was excited to pick his bicycle, his new two-wheeled adventure. We walked through the front doors of the store and Nico, walking through the outdoor section of the store, stopped in front of a lime green bicycle, sitting alongside the bike racks, as if someone had tried it and discarded it, forgetting to place it back on the rack. Nico straddled the seat, his feet meeting the ground at just the right spot. As chance would have it, this bike fit him perfectly. We let him pick out a helmet, a black and white one, and I made sure to find some training wheels that would accommodate a bike for an eight-year old. It was Nico's first time on a bike, and training wheels would be a necessity as he learned to ride. I wondered if he could ride without them and, deep down, I believed he could, and figured the training wheels would give us some time for him to learn. Before long, we were heading home, bike, helmet and training wheels tucked away safely in the trunk. Nico smiled the whole way home. He had his bike, and the smile that was spread across his face seemed to define his anticipation of joining his brother and sister on their bike riding excursions.

We had no more than two minutes from the time we pulled into the driveway that evening before Nico was requesting to ride his bike. It was dusk, and there wasn't much daylight left, but I decided to embrace his excitement and let him try his bike before we turned in for the night. I took the bicycle, along with the helmet, out of the trunk, and set it on the driveway.

Nico was excited. We attached the training wheels to the bike as Nico talked a mile a minute, his anticipation for riding mounting with each passing minute, the sun setting and working against us as we moved quickly. Finally, the training wheels were attached. We clipped Nico's helmet to his head and made our way up the street, with Nico's siblings following on their bikes. It was a perfect summer evening, the sun setting slowly, changing the sky into a variety of brilliant colors, the clouds perfectly outlined in shades of deep blue.

Nico mounted his bike and smiled. He pushed the pedals, riding alongside his siblings, and for a moment, I saw he was satisfied. He was riding his very new bike, on the sidewalk, his wish granted. After a minute or so, he stopped and looked at me. He looked into my eyes and said, "Mom, I don't want training wheels." My heart froze. I felt like I was punched in the stomach. I couldn't explain to him that the training wheels were the reason he was able to ride so easily, and without the training wheels, this would require balance, motor coordination, all things I was fairly certain would be challenging for him. This isn't entirely different than the way most parents feel the first time their children try something new, and, more specifically, take on the task of learning to ride a bike with two wheels alone. The difference here is that I was unsure of how receptive he would be to the change in the feel of the bike when the wheels were removed, and I hated, more than anything, thinking about his excitement leaving him, frustration instead takings its place. I wanted for him to feel the exhilaration and success I know he so badly craved. "Tomorrow," I replied, noticing the daylight fading too quickly to meet such demands this evening. Satisfied with this answer, Nico spent most of the remainder of our evening bike ride watching his brother and sister, who were riding without training wheels. I stood and watched, sad and happy at the same time. Why does everything, even bike riding, have to be a mountain climb for our son? I guess I hadn't accounted for the fact, or maybe I forgot, that our son already knows how to climb mountains better than anyone I know.

The next day we took the training wheels off of the bike and I took Nico on the sidewalk up the street to practice his bike riding. It was a beautiful, sunny, spring morning, a slight breeze enhancing the joyous feeling that comes with days early in this season. Nico sat on his bike as I held his seat from behind, ready to assist and guide him as he learned to ride without training wheels as a safety net. He looked at me and said, "No." I tried explaining to him that I was going to help him, but, not interested in hearing me explain my intentions, and eager to get started, Nico, again, repeated, "No," this time with a little more force. Hesitatingly, yet impressed with his resolve, I let go of the seat. Nico tried to push the pedals, but couldn't without losing balance, and he fell over. He stood back up, tried again, and fell over once more, landing hard on the sidewalk. His voice volume elevated, and he started yelling at the bike. I went to hold the seat again to try and help, and he yelled louder at me. "No!" I once again let go, my heart starting to break, and watched as he once again tried to push the pedals with his feet, yelling, "It's broken! Stupid bike is broken!" Tears slowly streaming down his cheeks, he tried to push the pedals with all of his might, and fell over. He stood up, picked up the bike, and threw it. He hid his face in his hands and cried. We went back down the street, me carrying the bike, Nico continuing to hide his face as he sobbed, silence enveloping us. I tried to think of a way I could help, but there wasn't. Here we were, faced with another challenge, and I was determined to help him accomplish his goal. I started to think of ways I could help. I spent the better part of that day researching adapted bikes, looking into programs in the area where I may be able to find a solution. A balance bike, maybe? Or a scooter? Maybe something that was easier to maneuver. I couldn't bare to watch him struggle again, and I wondered whether he would want to try after being so frustrated earlier that day.

The next morning, Nico came to me, requesting to ride his bike. I asked him if maybe he would want to put his training wheels back on his bike so that he would ride with his brother and sister once more, expecting him to agree to this compromise, at least for now. To my surprise, Nico responded, "No. No training wheels." Not knowing what to say in response, and with admiration for him and the fight within him, I joined Nico as we made our way back up the sidewalk, another spring morning in front of us. Nico sat on the bike once again. He pushed his feet on the pedals as hard as he could, and fell over. He tried once more, his frustration growing quicker than the day before, and before long, he was crying, frustrated that, for the second day in a row, he could not move on the bike. He yelled at me if I tried to hold the seat, much like the day before, and we found ourselves back home, Nico crying this time in the garage, yelling at me, "Why is the bike broken? Bike is broken!"

The next week continued like this, in much the same way. Except, with each passing day, Nico made small progress. First, he learned how to push the pedals forward. After he learned how to push the pedals, there was a lot of falling, and even more refusal of help. It was almost as if each day equated to a stronger will to do this on his own. If four days passed, Nico was four times more determined to accomplish his goal. There were a lot of cuts and scrapes, and each day, the mounting frustration was coupled with an increase in tears, yelling, and throwing. The bike was thrown, his helmet was thrown and scraped, and, one day, Nico became so overwhelmed that he ran in the house, crying, and hid for some time before emerging to play with his siblings. Nevertheless, there was small

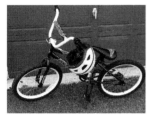 progress, every day. Watching from the sidelines, I found myself both amazed and wanting desperately to help, knowing that I couldn't. I would hide my tears from Nico as he worked through his frustration, powerless to help or stop it. All I could do was observe and be there to offer support. It is tough watching your child power through something they want more than anything, knowing only they can do it in the end.

About two weeks after his first bike ride, Nico had progressed to the point that he could sit on the bike and push the pedals a cycle or two before falling. On a spring morning in April, we made our way up the street once more, me, and my ever so determined eight-year old, with his lime green bicycle and black and white helmet. He mounted the bicycle. Not sure how much more he could take, and since his frustration had built so quickly the last few times we tried, I prepared for a quick turn around and figured we wouldn't be riding too long today. He put his right foot on the pedal, turned it, and then his left. His right, his left again. And again. He was riding his bike! He pushed a few turns before veering off into the grass. He turned his head over his right shoulder, his eyes smiling at me from just below the bottom of his helmet, his brown hair fringing his eyelashes. He did it! He proudly declared, "I'm riding!" For the first time since March, I saw smiles where tears were, and his bike and helmet were not thrown that day, but rather embraced. Our son. Our amazing, bike-riding son.

It was on this beautiful spring morning that Nico gave me the gift of determination. Watching my son take a challenge head-on, work through the tears, the anger, the soul-crushing frustration, and come out on the other side successful was one of the most inspiring things I've seen. Nico's lifestyle has made it so meeting and conquering challenges is part of his way of life. He knows how to take a challenge and make it his own, make it achievable, and experience success. Pain and threatening defeat are no match for him. Watching him work through this, on his own, without help, taught me the magic in tenacity. There are no easy answers sometimes. The things we often want most, in our hearts deepest desires, they require grit and a want so deep that it brings us to tears, to throwing things. The best thing we can do is never give up, to never lose the faith in ourselves, no matter how many scrapes, bumps and bruises come along with it. Watching him led me to reflect on my own approach to life. Do I have the courage to keep trying, to working through each step, until I achieve success? When I am met with a problem, do I retreat after I am met with frustration, or even disappointment? How much resolve do I have? From that day forward, when I am met with a challenge, I think of the green bicycle, and my son. His courage to get back on the bike, knowing that he could easily get hurt, and then trying again the next day. For not giving up, and for not giving in, thank you, Nico, for teaching me that nothing in this life is impossible.

THE RED CHAIRS

Writing a book about my son would feel incomplete if I didn't discuss the process of his diagnosis, of discovering an important and key part of the many things that make our son so special. This chapter is an important one for me to write. It holds a powerful message, a most precious gift.

Nico's journey to a diagnosis began when he was two years old. Noticing repetitive behaviors and some milestones in his development that took a little longer to reach, we called Early Intervention to schedule an initial evaluation. Three specialists came to our house in August of 2014. We answered a number of questions, and the specialists filled out checklists and worked one-on-one with Nico before they left for the day. Our follow-up appointment consisted of recommendations and discussions around some of the things we could do to help Nico, and many of the recommendations put forth centered around developing his communication. It wasn't long before we began speech therapy in our house. Twice a week a therapist would arrive with a basketful of toys, books, and papers, which she would use to work with Nico to help him develop both his expressive and receptive language skills. For months, her presence in our house became part of our norm, something to which we've become more accustomed in the years following his diagnosis.

A few months following his initial evaluation, our speech therapist mentioned that she noticed he didn't seem to answer her when she spoke to him. He would not turn when his name was called, and didn't seem interested in her when she tried to show him a new toy, or something fun. It was at this point that she suggested we see an audiologist. A hearing test would be a good starting point in determining if Nico had experienced some type of hearing loss in his young life. We called and made an appointment to have Nico's hearing tested, and a few months later, we found ourselves in the audiologists's office. Nico's hearing was tested, and the results showed that his hearing was considered unremarkable. While reviewing the results of the test, the audiologist suggested we meet with a local child development unit to further discuss Nico's developmental milestones and our concerns with his hearing, and so another appointment was made. It was at this appointment that the word "autism" was first introduced to us. We learned of a child psychologist in the area with whom we could speak who specialized in Autism. At this point in Nico's life, he was displaying some behaviors synonymous with Autism Spectrum Disorder (ASD), and the psychologist at the child development unit thought it would be beneficial for us to address some of these behaviors further. We made another phone call, and before long, had another appointment scheduled with another psychologist. His appointment with this psychologist was scheduled for the beginning of March, about two weeks before his 3rd birthday, and almost 8 months after our initial appointment with Early Intervention. Since our initial step on this journey with Early Intervention, up until and including this point, we had met with six different specialists and therapists. Our journey had only just begun. I remember thinking how odd it felt to meet and talk with so many people, to explain the same things over and over, and to leave each meeting in the same place we began, like going around and around in a wheel, with the hope of moving forward and somehow not moving forward at all.

Our appointment with the psychologist started to give us a clearer picture of what we had started to learn on our own. In the eight months since Nico's first evaluation with Early Intervention until now, while we were awaiting further professional insight and guidance, Nico was developing more and more behaviors indicative of ASD, giving us more to add to the conversations we would eventually have with the psychologist when the day of our appointment finally arrived. We met with this psychologist for three sessions, all of which were part of the diagnosis process. The initial session acted as a consultation, a time for the psychologist to get to know Nico and us. We brought a large pile of completed paperwork to this appointment, and spent a good amount of time talking about our son to the psychologist. The second appointment consisted of the screening itself, a chance for the psychologist to work one-on-one with Nico in order to collect any and all important data needed for her evaluation. This appointment took the longest, clocking in at just over three hours. During the third appointment, the psychologist reviewed her findings with us, his diagnosis, and any and all recommendations moving forward. All three sessions went well, and during the third appointment, where results were discussed, we learned that Nico had met all of the criteria for an ASD diagnosis, but would not yet be given one, as the build-up of fluid alleviated by the tubes surgically placed in his ears the fall prior may have caused Nico some trouble hearing, which in turn may have affected his development and his ability to assimilate to his environment. The passing of time would give us a much clearer understanding of Nico's milestones, behaviors, and the correct path to take moving forward. The recommendation of the psychologist moving forward was to begin wrap around services, where therapists would start meeting with us in the house for the following year to help Nico reach some key milestones in his development. Time, therefore, help us develop a deeper understanding of our son. Was it fluid build-up or ASD that was contributing to the path of his development? A prescription for these services, along with outpatient speech therapy, was given, as well as instructions to help us line up our medical benefits, and we were on our way. I came home that day feeling lost and more confused than ever. The plan was to follow these recommendations for the next 18 months, and when this time had passed, meet once again with the psychologist for another final evaluation. The journey for answers, for part of our son's truth, was long and involved. As we went through this process, our lives continued on as normal, with therapists and appointments becoming part of our norm. As our lives played out, so did the desire, the need for an answer to our questions, growing exponentially, week by week. It was like awaiting test results for 18 months. Imagine taking a final exam. The score on this exam determines every step you will ever take from that point moving forward. Your whole heart and soul will be affected by the results, and every step you take while awaiting these results may alter them. Our lives continued as normal, but my head never stopped. I remember sitting on the floor in the hallway outside of Nico's bedroom as he played a set of toy drums on the other side of the wall. The drumbeats were so rhythmic, and they lasted for almost 45 minutes nonstop. He had just turned three. I sat on my phone, researching autism symptoms behind tears as they welled in my eyes. I felt like I couldn't read about it too much. It was a club in which I was not yet a part, yet I knew, in my gut, that a membership card to this club was awaiting our son, awaiting us. I wanted so badly to belong somewhere with answers. Our time waiting on this journey wasn't all answerless questions and wondering, though. We worked with outpatient speech therapists, occupational therapists, and wraparound specialists in our house. We began to develop an understanding of acronyms and terms familiar to families of children with special needs. Our transition into this role didn't happen overnight, and not without thorough examination. As the months ticked on, Nico's behaviors aligned closer with ASD. As the hours in therapy added up, Nico continued to develop along the path set out for him, the destiny chosen for him. 18 months passed, and Nico grew 18 months older, accompanied the entire time by many new faces, practices, and meetings. Before I knew it, we were headed back to the psychologist. It was October of 2016. We were headed to the first of our three appointments, our consultation appointment, where we would talk with the psychologist and set dates for the following two appointments. This was the start of the end, as I saw it then. We were finally going to have an answer to the question that had been gnawing at my gut for the past two years. Would Nico be diagnosed with ASD?

We pulled up to the psychologist's building and I took Nico's hand as we walked up two flights of steps to the psychologist's office. My heart was in my throat, both nervousness and anticipation gripping me. The door swung open, and we were met with a dozen or so bright red chairs in the waiting room, pictures on the wall of children playing, a small set of

toys in the corner, and some magazines. We sat down in the set of three chairs clumped together along the far wall, and soon after we were asked to step into the room at the back of the office. As Nico played with toys on the floor, we talked with the psychologist about the progress Nico had made, the amazing things that make him who he is, the therapies Nico had completed, and the behaviors we had noted. After some time 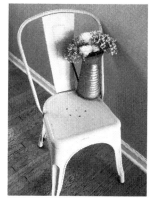 had passed, we left the psychologist's office, and waited for another two weeks for the most important appointment of all. It was time for his evaluation appointment. The time for answers was here.

Once again, we drove to the psychologist's office. Over our 18 months of waiting, one of the things we had found was that giving Nico names for people and places that were easy to differentiate was a helpful communication strategy. To Nico, the psychologist was known as the "Toy Doctor," as she had some fresh and new toys in her office that Nico enjoyed. During our initial consultation 18 months prior, he noted the toys, smiling as we played with them. From then on, we affectionately referred to her office as the office of the "Toy Doctor." As we neared the psychologist's office, we turned and said to Nico "Toy Doctor soon." He looked at us, and, in words as clear as day, he said, with a questioning tone to his voice, "The red chairs?" My jaw dropped. My head started spinning as I slowly began to understand that Nico was referring to the chairs in the office. I could not recollect if the chairs in the office were red, but I had a feeling that Nico did. We got out of the car and once again trekked across the parking lot to the office stairwell. We ascended the stairs and, as I pushed open the door to the waiting room, took a deep breath. The doors swung open, and there, before me, were a dozen or so red chairs. I stopped, frozen. The red chairs. How did he remember? This may have been the first time his visual memory astounded me, but it wouldn't be the last.

The appointment played out as I understood it would. Nico went with the psychologist into her office while we waited in the ever fateful red chairs. After about three hours, the psychologist appeared from the back room and thanked us for coming. She said she would meet with us in two weeks to discuss her results. More waiting. The day of our third and final appointment came. I sat in those red chairs, along with my husband Paul, as we waited for our turn to meet with the psychologist in the small room in the corner. The door to her office finally opened, her requesting us to join her. Nico played with toys on the floor as Paul and I sat in chairs across from her, chairs that, as fate would have it, were red. She began to talk with us about her findings, the diagnostics, the details of their three hours together during his appointment a few weeks prior, his behaviors and things that impressed her and made her smile, things she noted, as well as a number of other details of their playdate before saying the words I can still hear in intonation, weight, and importance: "I see no reason to wait any longer. Your son meets the criteria for an Autism Spectrum Disorder diagnosis," she said softly, pausing after, looking at us, awaiting a reaction. Not completely taken aback and almost relieved in a sense to know part of my son's truth, I, armed with what I thought was a good understanding of the situation, listened as she proceeded to explain her findings and his diagnosis further. She clarified everything, talking with us in great detail, and concluded our appointment that day by reviewing with us specific recommendations moving forward, as well as resources we could use as we set out on this new journey in parenthood. It was as if someone had wiped the blurry film away from my eyes. I looked at my son. I knew his truth. For the first time in a long time, I could see my son. I was able to SEE MY SON. I packed up our things, almost numb, took Nico's hand, and walked past those red chairs, to the stairwell, and eventually to the car. As we drove away, I realized that, from that point forward, our lives would be different. And yet, somehow, it felt as though we were on the road on which we had been destined to travel all along.

The story of Nico's diagnosis is important. It gave to us, inarguably, one of the most precious and valuable gifts of all. Walking into the waiting room that day, seeing those red chairs, the red chairs my son had already predicted, awakened a feeling in me. It dawned on me that day that we were walking into where we were meant to be. It felt right, though I felt I wanted to run away when our son's diagnosis was revealed to us that day, the path before us set, scary, new, and unpredictable. The roads before us are paved the way they are for a reason. They are laid before us in a way that calls to the destiny in all of us. More importantly, knowing that part of this journey to our destiny may be blurry at times, revealing amazing things along the way, when the time is right. That day, in the psychologist's office, my son, his truth, all of it amazing, was revealed to me. That road, that part of the path, no longer blurry, but instead crystal clear. Resisting the journey, ignoring signs of one's destiny, they only lead to more complexities, more blur. That day, we learned the importance of accepting where you are meant to be, where the roads are meant to take us. Those red chairs, that feeling in my heart, it was the last step in a series of steps, an awakening of sorts. All of the signs confirmed our road was the right one. Why we were chosen for this journey, I will never know. I'm not sure I need to. One thing is for certain-my son has taught me that resisting who you were meant to be, fighting to not see where you are clearly, it stops you from your, "ah ha!" moment. It stops you from finding your red chairs, your sign, the undeniable truth laying before you. The clues that unfold day to day, year to year, that show you that you are fulfilling your destiny. Thanks to Nico, I now understand, truly, the gift of accepting your truth, your path, and realizing the amazing things that await when you truly see, live, and embrace the life that was meant for

DANA BAUER

you

SAYING GOODBYE

Focusing on the gifts Nico has given us in his life so far and the absolute joy that is parenting our remarkable son, this book has a positive theme, an uplifting vibe, and it is my hope that our son's story brings inspiration to anyone reading this book, and that his life brings light to the lives of others. This chapter, though it will do the same, will be presented from a different angle. This chapter will take a look at denial. No one life is void of challenges or struggles. It is in these times that acceptance becomes imperative, because, without it, one cannot fully move on, fully grow. This chapter will focus on the time I had to say goodbye.

Nico's diagnosis, discussed in the previous chapter, was one of the most poignant and important moments in his life. With this new diagnosis, his life would set out on a different course than what was initially expected. Though not altogether surprising, I do remember a number of feelings that came over me that October day in the psychologist's office. These feelings, they would become very familiar to me. They would become part of me, as Nico's mom, as his temporary voice until he could find his own, as the captain of this new ship upon which we were thrust. These feelings, these thoughts, they would become a narrative that would play out over and over again, a cycle in my head, and it was at this time that my perspective narrowed. I learned a survival mechanism: I started seeing life and living life with conveniently blurred lenses. Focusing on the positive is something most of us do, most of us strive for each day. We are told to look at the the bright side, to embrace changes and be flexible. We are told to look at the glass as half full, and to not sweat the small stuff. These are powerful messages by which to live, and doing these things can certainly make the tough times easier. They are not bad messages to embrace by any means. The problem arises when you become afraid to take off these lenses and see clearly.

You are so afraid to see certain aspects of a situation that you purposely make them blurry so that you cannot see them clearly. What if they are dangerous? What if they are scary? You will do anything to avoid it, even when it means you can't grasp an all-encompassing view imperative to growth. Sometimes, seeing things clearly allows you to see the whole picture, and so avoiding some details of the big picture at all costs, keeping certain aspects of your life blurred out, may be temporarily comfortable, but it is not healthy. It is not positive, and it can do more harm than good. It was on this day that I made the decision to keep my blurred lenses on, and I learned, over time, that I, too, was missing the bigger picture.

I went home the day of the appointment numb. I did not know what to say. I was made aware of an entirely new reality for our son, for our family. I didn't know what to do with this news. I don't mean that metaphorically. I truly did not know what to do with what was just handed to me. I came home, called my parents and my husband's parents, and told them what we learned. I made another phone call to our local Early Intervention office, and that was it. There was no ceremony, or some major announcement, some monumental Oscar- winning music to signify to me whether this was the beginning or the end of something new. There was not a giant shift in the course of my life. There was nothing notably abnormal about that day. It carried on in just the same way the other days in my life did. It was a Thursday. I went to work the next day, and the weeks that followed. My life, Nico's life, my husband's life, and our family's life carried on as it would have without that appointment. When this happens, when you're handed this new set of cards, one needs time to process. Without that time, things happen, like what happened to me. I went through the motions of my day-to-day, a giant void growing inside. It was almost an out-of-body experience. I was expected to carry on, to live as I always had, but I did not have time to stop. I did not have time to process. I did not have time to cry. I did not have time to write. I did not have time to exercise, to draw, to express all I was feeling. I had to carry on, in real time, while trying to grapple with everything. I became numb, looking for ways to distract myself. The more normal things were, the more in control I was. This is how my attempt to only see what I wanted, to stay where things were easy and smooth, started. I began painting rooms in my house, and rearranging furniture. I had bursts of creative energy, and, in what little downtime I had, would find new projects to take on, painting my interior doors and walls dark colors, my exterior garage doors and front door dark. Subconsciously, painting became a distraction, and the dark colors, almost symbolic, representing feelings growing inside me that I conveniently chose to ignore. Friends and family, their lives continued on, and ours did, too, although I felt as though I was in a race, day to night, night to day, and my only goal was to avoid stopping for too long. It was in stopping that I could not avoid certain details of my son's life, of our life as a family, and I desperately wanted to see only what I wanted to see. The world expected me to act as if there was nothing new in our lives, nothing major or large, as if I didn't have this new journey to navigate, to understand. With each passing day, the small reality inside me, the one I knew I needed to face, kept growing, the scary parts and the parts that weighed heavily on me, they beckoned me to look at them, to understand them, to study them. I reacted with resistance. I kept covering these calls with projects, with work, with distractions. I started losing sleep, I stopped eating, but I kept going, I kept running. Avoiding the reality, avoiding the pit in my stomach that kept growing. It is single handedly the hardest thing in the world to try and carry on, when the world and friends and family expect you to do so, and you, yourself, have to try, all the while, carrying something deep. Certain details of the big picture, becoming slowly more recognizable, and you busying yourself more because you are not ready to stop and see them. And then, one day, you run out of places to go. You've distracted yourself in every way imaginable, and you've run out of time. The time has come for you to acknowledge all aspects of your life or a situation, for they allow you to see the bigger picture, the picture as a whole. You must face it head on, with all of the courage you can muster, even though you are shaking with fear. You stiffen your shoulders, you hold your head up high, and you take it. You stop running, and you squint your eyes to see what you've been trying to outrun. Your feet may be swept out from under you as you are enveloped in what you have been trying to avoid. And then, a strange thing happens. After spending some time there, things slowly coming into focus, you realize there is peace there, and beauty there, too. In fact, things you've been avoiding, the things you now see clearly, are breathtaking. They are exciting and new and fresh. And in seeing them, you are finally able to see the forest through the trees. You see the bigger picture, and you develop a deep and complete understanding because you've allowed yourself to see everything, to take it all in. Not doing this would stop us from fully enjoying everything there is to enjoy. It wouldn't be fair, and you may miss out on some of the best and most wonderful things. Most people call this denial. To me, denial was the worst of all things. How could I truly enjoy who my son is if I kept painting things, if I kept doing projects, if I kept ignoring my son's truth, all of it, and avoided seeing the big picture? Seeing my incredible son in his entirety? I approached nobody else in my life this way. I experienced each member of my family and friend circle completely, understanding all of them, all of their truths. It was time for me to take off my lenses.

And so it came to be. One night, as I was putting my son to bed, the seed of reality became too big. I adjusted Nico's blanket around his shoulders, gently tucking him in. I bent down to give him a kiss, like usual, and walked to the door, shutting it softly behind me. And I stood, in the hallway, in the dark, the night-light from the quiet upstairs hallway shining just enough to let me see. And it dawned on me. This small glimmer of light. It was all I needed to guide me. My son's beautiful face, his charisma, his amazing heart and soul. I stiffened my shoulders, I held my head high, and I took a deep breath. It was time to say goodbye, and it was time to say hello. I took off my lenses.

I turned around, and quietly opened the door to his bedroom. I looked at him, sleeping, peacefully in his bed. I softly tiptoed to the side of his bed, crouched down, his breathing soft in front of my face. "Don't leave me, Nico." I said to him. "I'm sure going to miss you. I'm going to miss what I thought was. I'm going to miss my dreams I had for you. But, man, am I sure excited to see where you take me. What you teach me. I am so happy to be your mother. Your mother. You, my beautiful, sweet, guy. Goodbye...." And I cried, silently, into my arm. I cried, I sobbed silently, for what seemed like forever. And I now moved from a crouching position, to a cuddled up sitting position on the floor, curled into a ball. I cried for what I thought was going to be. I cried for the first almost four years, and how that life, those thoughts, they would be different now. My body, heavy with pain, lay still, with tears staining my face, for a long time. Just me, Nico, and the soft dark of evening, all of the details I had been ignoring becoming crystal clear. And when a great deal of time passed, I sat up. I wiped my face, and I turned and looked at my son. For the first time in months I was able to actually look at my son. I was able to see him, and not what I thought would be. It was spectacular, better than anything I previously thought. How lucky I am, I thought. Look at this amazing child. How wonderful, and how great he is. "I am so lucky to be your mom. I love you," I whispered into his ear. I kissed him once more and I walked out of the room, closing the door silently behind me, closing the door on what I thought was going to be, and moving into the hallway, a new sense of understanding about me, the glimmer of light all I needed at the time to see clearly all that my son is, and all of the amazing parts of him.

Dealing with pain, with unmet expectations, with sadness, grief, and surprises, they are a part of life, they are a part of us all. Thanks to Nico, I have been given a gift. The gift that allows me to see all of the details, how to acknowledge them, how to see them as an important part of the bigger picture and not the whole picture. Seeing things for all they are is an important aspect of appreciating them, of celebrating them and their truth, and this is imperative to growth. My son has given me the ability to face life with an entirely new perspective. I often wonder where I would be without him to help me understand this. I wonder what other details in life I might be missing if I hadn't learned how to take off my blurred lenses. He is my light. He is my best teacher, and I am forever grateful for him.

A DECK DOOR, AND THE START OF SOMETHING NEW

Most people have many questions for me in regards to raising a child diagnosed with ASD. The most common inquiries I receive are related, in some way, to how and when we first "knew." People most often ask how old our son was when he was diagnosed, what it is like living with someone as wonderful as Nico, and where specialists think Nico will be in the years to come. To answer these questions, I would first need to take you both to the past and to the future. Both of these destinations hold answers, though one is more definitive, while the other wildly and excitedly unpredictable.

Nico's childhood began like any other, with a newborn phase unremarkable, developmentally right on track. My beautiful, blue eyed baby was, and still is, the light of my life. As his babyhood progressed on, he almost seemed to veer off on his own road, his own tangent. Crawling looked different for Nico than my other children, with Nico crawling with one leg and standing with the other, simultaneously. Words followed their own path, as well. Nico did not develop a vocabulary as quickly as our other children, nor did he every learn to use a sippy cup. He only preferred the same solid foods, and sleep was difficult for him. None of these milestones stood out as anything remarkable, but they were notable. It was in these milestones that we unknowingly began walking down a new path, a journey on a road parallel to the one that we had anticipated, on the one we had started when Nico was born in 2012. For a long time, we straddled both of these paths, one running right beside the other. Some days were spent on one path, but I couldn't help but feel that I wanted to try this other path. This new path that I had discovered next to the original looked intriguing and comforting and right in some way. In 2014, our family attended a wedding in Maine for my cousin. It was this trip that started to define this second path for us.

Maine is a beautiful state, especially in the summer. The leaves are blanketed in green, the air smelling of summer in the country at its finest, with water and shores dotted with large stones, lighthouses spotted along the coast. My aunt's family owns a house in Maine, situated along a beautiful river, nestled among the trees, settled at the end of a gravel road. It is picturesque and beautiful, something out of a novel. My cousin settled on Bar Harbor for her wedding, and so we enjoyed a week with family at my aunt's house. Most days

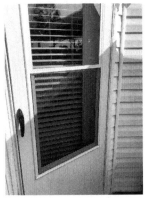 during our week there, when not preoccupied with a myriad of wedding preparations, were spent swimming, with relaxing afternoons on the couch in the family room, or trips to the local state parks, and evenings on the house deck with family. Lobster, corn, good food, and great memories with family would occupy my memory when I think of this trip. Nestled in along with these memories would be the first definitive step in our autism journey-the moment we "knew," if I were to call it this.

An evening dinner turned into time with family surrounding a fire outside of my aunt's house. The sun, pink and almost purple, a beautiful backdrop to our evening. My cousin's children and a few of my children played in the grass alongside the house while the adults sat around the fire pit next the deck, the river running smoothly in the background. I would occasionally look around to do a quick "head count," keeping an eye on my children as they played with their cousins in the grass. One time, when looking up, I noticed that Nico was missing. Not overly concerned, I stood up and made my way to the side yard, looking around a bit closer, with still no signs of Nico. I heard a tapping noise on the deck, and as I turned to the direction of this sound, saw our son. He was standing on the deck, pulling open the wooden screen door and slamming it closed, over and over again, repeatedly. Have you ever had a moment when something in plain sight becomes clear? When an answer for which you have been seeking almost appears out of nowhere, but not out of nowhere at all? It was this moment, with the deck door, where we first used the word "autism." It was here that our journey officially started.

Phone calls and doctors appointments led us to the diagnosis. But Nico's journey did not stop there. In fact, it had just begun. Because of this deck door, because of this beginning, we set out on a new course. Our son was about to open our eyes to things we never would have known or experienced. It is because of him that I have had privileges beyond measure, it is because of him that we were invited into a secret and special world.

Nico is the reason that my family and I participate in parades in cities around our town. My children are able to ride on floats because of him. Because of Nico, I have had the utmost privilege of meeting everyday heroes, people who spend their lives making things better for others. Nico is to thank for growing our family. We have specialists and therapists who have spent every week alongside us, watching our children grow, along with Nico. It is because of Nico that we've met professional dog trainers, we've been featured on social media pages of professional sports teams and multiplatinum bands. We've become involved with people in other states, walking roads we never would've seen if it weren't for our son. We have met families whose paths we wouldn't have crossed otherwise. The families, these people, they are incredible people. Having a child with special needs means you are invited into a sort of "club." A group of people who live each day with their hearts raw. There is an amazing sweetness and sincerity around people who know how it feels to be grateful for the smallest things, for the tribe you find in others. There is something magical about surrounding yourself with people who don't have time to busy themselves with trivial matters, or pretentious ambitions. People who live truly inspirational lives. Some people I consider to be good friends now-their human resumes consist of giving their life savings to make the lives of special needs children better, they give up positions of authority to others for the betterment of all. Many of my friends I've met on my journey as Nico's mother are people who make daily, selfless sacrifices and live almost impossible truths. I sometimes think about the amazing things our family has experienced, and the incredible people we've met, all because of Nico. I would like to tell you that I have an end to this story, but the story, Nico's story, is not done yet. I have no idea where this journey will take us. It is exciting and thrilling when you think about the many things our son's life has introduced us to. The deck door in Maine-it was the start of something new. What an incredible, amazing journey it has been so far. Thank you for opening the door and inviting us to journey with you, Nico.

SUMMER DAYS

The pool-our neighborhood pool, to be exact. A favorite destination of ours on hot, summer days in Pennsylvania. Many of our friends meet at the pool for some relaxation, fun, and companionship. The snack bar is always open, music playing in the speakers affixed to the lights surrounding the pool, lifeguards watching from high above in their chairs. Summer afternoons spent at the pool are our favorites.

One day in mid July, the sun and heat at their most extreme, we packed our pool bag for an afternoon of sun and fun. I made sure to pack towels, juice boxes, diving sticks, pool floats, and, of course, goggles, as well as water guns and toy watering cans. Nico, as well as my other children, have their preferred pool toys, and ensuring I have them packed with us always guarantees our times at the pool are extra fun for everyone. Arriving at the pool without our second son's diving sticks that he uses in competitions with his friends, or without my daughter's goggles she uses when diving in the deep end, without our other son's pool float, or without Nico's watering can, which he enjoys using to spray water in small streams endlessly, would surely end in disappointment.

The bag packed, and sunscreen applied, we headed to the car. The sun beat down on us as we packed the car, and we were off. As we pulled into the gravel parking lot, it quickly became apparent that many other members of the pool had the same idea as us on this scorching day. The pool was crowded, many people enjoying the cool water, a relief from the heat.

We found a pool chair close to the shallow end of the pool on which to place our things. I emptied the towels and sunscreen out of the bag to make it easier for the children to find their pool toys, all of which had found a home on the bottom of the bag. The floats were clipped onto our youngest children, and goggles placed on their faces. Nico grabbed his watering can and announced he was ready to join the others in the pool. I pulled my windswept hair out of my eyes into a messy ponytail. Four excited children at the pool and a hot summer afternoon leaves very little room for vanity. I reached into the pool bag to grab sunscreen, my final step before I, too, was ready to join the others, and looked up. Nico was looking at me, his green eyes soft. He was smiling out of the corner of his mouth. "Hi, Sweet Guy," I said to him. He didn't break eye contact as he replied, "Mom, you're beautiful." He leaned in to give me a long kiss. He waited for me to finish getting myself ready for an afternoon in the water, and we walked, hand in hand, to the side of the pool.

Nico sees the many things this world has to offer with purity, without bias, without the negative, judgmental filter though what most of us see. He sees things in their rawest form. The day he looked at me at the pool and said the words he did was profound. It was moving. Most of us spend hours, whether consciously or subconsciously, taking life's most simple joys or pleasures, and come at them with a bias. That giant piece of cake? Yes, it is good, but it is loaded with calories. The waves at the beach? Sure, they are fun, but what about sharks? How about that movie you've been waiting to see for so long? Yes, it is in theaters, with only a week or so left, but who wants to wait in the lobby with a bunch of screaming children on a Friday or Saturday night? And the popcorn and candy? Overpriced. The veil though which we see this world, for most of us, is tinted grey. It is layers deep, with each layer carrying a different experience or feeling that eventually clouds the way we see things. My son has given me the ability to remove this veil. The ability to see things as they are, for what they are. When he looked at me and said the words he did, it was because he saw beauty. Not messy hair, dark roots peeking through the blonde, wrinkled lines around my eyes and forehead, or my lack of makeup. These are all layers of my veil, how I see myself, how I perceive how I had "failed" to fill the expectation of a fun, young mom at the pool. He saw me. Raw.

No bias. This gift, to recognize how many things around us, are beautiful, exciting or special, simply because they are, is a gift. The $5 hanging basket of flowers in my front yard, those pink blooms now stop me in my tracks. No longer do I think about the dying flowers in the basket, or how I wanted to buy the $25 basket. I now see vibrant pink, a beautiful color, made even more so against the grass behind it. If you catch me playing in the snow with my children on a blustery winter day, it is because I've been given a gift. The snow is beautiful. It is fun to build ramps, and snowmen, complete with scarves and a carrot nose. I no longer notice how cold it is, or how challenging it is to keep track of snow gear for four young people. I've been taught how to remove my veil, to see the truth, it's simplicity and beauty overwhelming. Thank you, Nico. I hope I never remember how to put it back on.

A FIRE HALL AND ICE

In the summer of 2019, my husband and I discussed potentially starting Nico in an extracurricular sport of some kind. He was seven years old and did not have any extracurricular activities of his own, unless you count attending his sister's football games and his brother's soccer games as extracurricular activities. We knew of some adapted sports in our area-horseback riding lessons and the Miracle League Baseball, to be exact. The Miracle League has two fields near us, one used for a season that had already started, and another, which was not slated to open until the following year, thus striking the idea of baseball off of the list, at least for the time being. Horseback riding lessons also peaked our interest, but we knew that this would be more therapeutic than extracurricular, and, with some research, we learned of a special needs hockey association in our area. I called the coach in late July, who told me that the new season would soon be starting. We would need to attend sign-ups, which were scheduled at a local fire hall at the beginning of August. He explained a little about the program before our phone conversation ended. I was excited and intrigued. Ice hockey-I never pictured myself being a "hockey mom." Nobody in my family played the sport growing up, and neither did my friends. I guess we would see what the meeting held for us. Would this be a good fit for Nico? For our family?

The beginning of August came, and we found ourselves outside of the local fire hall where the meeting was being held. As we exited the car, I had feelings of butterflies in my stomach. I knew, as I looked at the doors to the fire hall, that I was about to enter uncharted waters. I had no idea what to expect, and my mind and heart were simultaneously flooded with doubt, questions, and hope.

We walked into the fire hall that afternoon, and what I saw before me astounded me. On the left were piles of hockey equipment. Helmets, equipment bags, skates, gloves, shin guards. Multiple piles of equipment, piled as high as my knees. In front of us were two long, white tables set up with women sitting at them, piles of papers neatly organized in front of them. The line forming at the end of these tables told me this was where we needed to be, and so we walked over and took our place at the end of the line. As I waited, I continued to scan the room. Chairs were set up in the front of the room, a table with trophies on it, a red ice hockey jersey, and other paraphernalia. A television was set up next to the table, and a number of adults were wandering around the room, all of whom were proudly adorned with the team name. It was finally our turn at the table. The woman at the table asked us about Nico and got some information about him before turning to me and telling me to make our way over the equipment area. I turned to face it, and as we began walking across the tile floor to what seemed like the endless piles of equipment, a man walked over to us. He introduced himself, and began helping us fill an equipment bag with all of the equipment Nico

would need on the ice. I began to realize that this equipment was donated, and a strong wave of humility and gratefulness washed over me. After filling our equiment bag, we walked to

 the front of the room, where we found chairs on which to sit. Parents, I presumed at the time, of other hockey players filled in around me, as the head coach walked across the front of the room. He proceeded to provide the parents with information about the organization and the hockey season. After he finished speaking, we were treated to a small video presentation about the program before leaving for the day. We pulled out of the parking lot after our meeting at the fire hall with so many unanswered questions. Was Nico going to be able to tolerate skates? A neck guard? How will the coaches know to take things slow, to use visuals? If he falls once, will he forever associate the sport with the pain of a fall on the ice? What if he is the only child struggling? What if he never gets it? Never once did I think a single thought that day that would eventually become a reality for us.

The season began in September. The very first practice, I took Nico by myself. I took a deep breath as I dressed him prior to the start of practice. Anticipating a meltdown or resistance to the equipment, I took things slow. To my surprise, there was no resistance at all, but instead, Nico, with all of his equipment on, his chest pad and shoulder pads making his arms bulge, flexed his muscles, and from behind his mask on his helmet, through a half crooked smile, said, "I'm a big hockey guy." I smiled. Pleasantly surprised, I took his hand and led him to the ice. I found him a walker made of PVC pipe and I guided him as he stepped on the ice for the first time, smiling at me as he went.

Three weeks of practice passed, and Nico went from stepping onto the ice to skating fairly quickly, still with the walker. Practices for Nico were a somewhat serious affair. On the ice, it appeared that Nico was alone, he and the ice in a partnership of sorts, accompanied only by his skates and his equipment. He paid no attention to any of the other players or coaches, but instead focused on how to move his legs in such a way that he glided easier on the ice. His attention was set on holding onto the walker, and the angle at which his skates pointed, how his helmet sat in such a way that he could see through the mask, and how to adjust the angle of his neck so that the neck guard ideally only lightly brushed against his skin. It was Nico and the Ice. A perfect match. A surprising love story, one developing before my very eyes. I spent each of these three practices with tears forming in my eyes. My son...he was surprising me. I was slowly rewriting a book on my son, one that was written, at least in my head, in stone, by me. I was wrong. And I loved watching him prove me so.

During his fourth week of practice, Nico, for the first time, ditched the walker. Now, again, it was Nico and the Ice, alone. Only this time, there was intense attention paid to how to move without the walker, without anything on which to balance. Nico, paying no attention to anyone around him, would watch his feet, look up at the ice, look back down, move his arms, slowly, until he was able to shimmy a few feet across the ice. I started to slowly realize the meaning of and weight behind the statement, "You can do anything you set your mind to." Our son was ice skating, by himself, even if it was a foot or so.

As the season progressed, and each practice came to pass, Nico progressed by leaps and bounds, each practice bringing something new to his repertoire, and, incidentally, bringing me to tears. I was thrilled to learn that I knew nothing about my son and his capabilities, and I've never been more happy to be proven wrong in my life.

This hockey experience, one which we currently still enjoy, taught me an amazingly powerful lesson. Yes, the old adage, "You can do anything you set your mind to," rings clear and true, but the gift goes much deeper here. Watching Nico on the ice taught me the importance and benefits to an open mind and heart. So many doctors, therapists, teachers, specialists, parents, support groups, they've tried to paint a picture for us, they've tried to tell us all about our son. Articles, magazines, blog posts, they think they have the answers, too. Watching Nico on the ice taught me that he, and he alone, has the answers. Much like our other children, Nico's accomplishments and setbacks will be played out over the course of his life. In this sense, he is no different than anyone else, and I am so glad he proved me and my expectations about hockey wrong. Our son is capable of absolutely incredible things. I watched him prove this over many weeks of ice hockey, a sport I was sure he could never do. The word, "never." It should never be in any of our vocabularies, and especially not in mine.With an open mind, and an open heart, every opportunity that falls before us is a gift, a chance to show ourselves and others of what we are truly capable. Nobody can write the books on my son better than he can. Hockey is but one chapter, a blank slate lying before him, and an open mind and heart for all of those in the audience. Thank you for teaching me to watch you, Nico. For showing me how much I don't know, for showing me how much you do know, and for showing me how to appreciate the journey, with all of its twists, turns.....and ice.

COURAGE IN A DOG

It is often said that a dog is a man's best friend. A few years ago, our son took to elopement. In regards to those with an ASD diagnosis "elopement" is common, and at times, can be considered worrisome. When most people think of eloping, they think of people taking off without any prior indication to get married. In regards to ASD "elopement," means the same thing, minus the marriage part. Nico starting "eloping" when he was three years old. Certain things, with with no prediction, would grab Nico's attention. A curious Halloween decoration, for instance, used to be perched on the top storage shelf in the garage, its orange and purple ribbons peeking out in such a way that the colors stood out against the other black storage bins. This decoration was, at one time, fascinating to Nico, enough so that he did, at one time, walk out to the garage without us knowing in order to study it from afar. Another time, it was the bricks atop the garage entryway, laid in a circular motion.There was always a worry in the pit of my stomach that Nico would one day try to touch or find these objects, and would accidentally hurt himself. A worry about young children doing things to hurt themselves is a common theme of parenthood. We have electric plug covers, and stove covers, and toilet seat locks. There are no pieces of safety equipment to help with elopement, and we were always worried that Nico would one day get himself into an accidental predicament.

One sunny summer afternoon, I noticed that Nico was missing from the toy room. Anxiety and panic mounting, I began calling for Nico, searching each room of our house, leaving no closet or under bed storage area unchecked. I couldn't find Nico. My heart began to beat faster, and steadily increasing, with tears welling in my eyes. I had read about elopement, heard stories of parents in this same situation. The stories always began much like this afternoon. Was this one of those times? Had he eloped?

Is he ok? As fear gripped me tighter around the throat, I heard my doorbell ring. My neighbor was waiting for me. "Nico is throwing rocks in our yard," he said, softly, with kindness and patience in his voice. "Oh, thank God," I replied, relieved. I ran outside, shoeless, desperate to find him. "We will clean up the rocks. I am so sorry," I told my neighbor. He looked at me with a look that I would describe as both sympathetic and apologetic, for I was not prepared what I would find when I finally did make it to his yard. Nico really enjoyed playing with our neighbor's dog, a big, black Goldendoodle. It wasn't uncommon for Nico to spend time playing with this dog and his toys while our other children were playing on the swings in our backyard, or jumping on the trampoline. Today was no different in this regard. I saw Nico, standing in my neighbor's backyard, river rock strewn around him on their patio, in their grass, on their outdoor furniture. Nico was playing a game of fetch with their dog that afternoon, the river rock being the toys he used. I stopped in my tracks, realizing quickly that this was more than a few rocks being tossed playfully in the air. I assessed the scene. There were river rocks everywhere. My neighbor's patio furniture was littered with them, their patio covered in them, their yard taken over by them. After ensuring Nico was not hurt, my only sense of relief coming in this station that our son was, indeed, safe, I turned to my neighbor, and assured him that I would help clean up the rock. Our neighbor, with much grace and patience, replied, understandingly, "It is ok. I'm just glad he is ok." I took Nico back into the house and spent the next three hours in my neighbor's backyard, cleaning up rock, assessing our neighbor's patio, furniture, and outdoor space for damage. The rest of the day had me on edge. I was worried. How do I keep Nico safe? I was out of ideas, exhausted and worried.

The next day, I was surfing the web for ideas to help us when I stumbled upon a company called K9's for Kids. I clicked on the name of the website and read about the program and services they provided. I was hooked instantly. A service dog-the perfect answer! I read a number of stories and testimonials on the website, and found a number of them sharing about times their child's dog helped find their child when he or she went missing. The dogs were trained to find their child. They were trained to do other things as well, and the program highlighted the many ways it could and would be catered to Nico's exact needs. I called the contact number found on the website and spoke to the trainer in charge of the program. He explained to me a little about what it entailed, and asked me if I'd like to attend a training session to see the program before committing. From this phone call, I learned that these dogs, and the training associated with them, come with a hefty price tag, but the benefits were tremendous. We attended our first training session, outdoors, in a local park, on a warm September afternoon. I was brought to tears when I saw the dogs tracking their "boys," their children. The dogs would bark as the children, guided by a dog, simulated elopement. The dogs used scent to track their boys, finding them, even when the boys would hide far away in the simulation. Elopement would be no longer. Our son would be safe, my worries comforted. I spoke with the trainer after the session, and he explained to me some examples of fundraising ideas to try, as well as the timeline for how and when we would not only get a puppy, but participate in and complete the training program. It would last a little over a year, with training taking place every week, for 2 hours or so, outside, in any and all elements He explained that they train in all weather, and that we would need to commit to the program in order for our dog to graduate. Thinking of my son's happiness, safety, and the benefits of him having such a companion, my excitement grew. We began to plan and organize fundraisers when I arrived home that day, and within one month, we had enough money raised for Nico's dog. We received Jake late that following October and began training in January.

During our first week of training I was nervous and intimidated. Jake, our German Shepherd Dog, was now 10 weeks old, and getting bigger by the hour. All black, he was a beautiful puppy who I knew would grow into a powerful dog. I didn't know what to do. Our trainer helped show me how to handle him, as well as some other training strategies, and he

showed me how to help him bond with Nico. Nico would be the only one to feed him, and we spent hours at home that first week practicing some of the bonding techniques and hand-ling techniques we were taught during our first morning train- 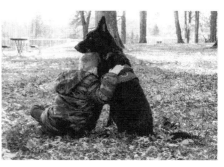 ing. I went home after our first session with a small seed of confidence. I had stepped way out of my comfort zone.

With each passing week, challenges arose, and I had to find my confidence, my strength, to help make Jake's training go as smoothly as possible. One time, while practicing obedience, I called for Jake to come to me. "Here," I yelled, as forcefully as I could, in a voice I thought mimicked that of the alpha in the situation. Our trainer, unimpressed with my voice, yelled back, "Is that a command or request?" "A command," I replied, know-ing what was coming in response. "Then get your voice to sound like it," said our trainer, smiling at me. This statement, this ex-perience, still resinates deeply within me. It was, at this moment, I realized that this dog training experience was about far more than finding a companion for my son, that it carried a weight far heavier than finding a solution to Nico's elopement.

It was in our dog training experience that Nico gave me an important gift. He helped me become the person I always wanted to be. It was about me learning, along with Jake, to protect Nico. I had to find my voice, my confidence in myself as a dog handler, and alongside this, my confidence and my place in my role all of this. This journey, one of a special needs parent, it isn't for the weak, the faint in voice and heart. It is for the strong. It requires a command of presence, a demand for the best life for your child, a "stop-at-nothing" attitude. It requires of me, it demands of me at times, to dig deep, evolve, and grow. Nico's elopement brought us to dog training, and dog training brought me into this sense of self, this growing process. It forced me to find my voice, to leave my old self behind, to morph, almost, into someone whose voice, as our trainer said that day, "sounds like it." My voice, my self-"sounding" like strength and confidence. Challenges in life force us to do one of two things-evolve and grow, and rise to the occasion, or shrivel and shrink, succumbing to what is presented to us. Dog training helped develop the fight in me. When faced with a challenge during our year of training, I was expected to find a solution. I was expected to find the strength and confidence to overcome it so that I could teach Nico the techniques necessary to succeed and eventually have Jake graduate from the program. If I was walking Jake on his leash and he began pulling me, I had to find my strong voice and take the lead. When our training session had ended a year later, I was ready. Jake was ready. Nico was ready. Our family was ready. We had a year to grow, to develop, to graduate, ready to take on any of the challenges that lay before us. Jake, our dog, is now Nico's best companion, a wonderful friend, and an excellent protector. To me, he is a constant reminder of where I was, and where I am now. I often affectionately say that Nico has turned me into the person I always wanted to be. I guess I should offer gratitude to Jake, too, who helped give me the courage to get there.

MY SON AND A CONGA LINE

Every year, the Parent Teacher Association at the primary school in our school district hosts a school dance. The dance is separated so that grades in the school attend the dance on separate days. It is run after school one day in the early spring, and lasts for about an hour. It is a wonderful time for the children, and it gives them something to which they can look forward as the long days of winter make their transition to spring. The dance itself is very low key. A DJ sets up his equipment in the gym, the lights are dimmed, and a number of parents stand around and chaperone as the children dance, run, talk, and laugh for an hour. It is a great time for our children to join together in fun. Nico attended this dance in both first and second grade. It was during this dance, during Nico's second grade year, that Nico showed me what courage looks like.

I arrived at the school that day at 3:45, right as the dance was beginning. I walked into the school and around the corner, where the cafeteria awaited me, just a few feet ahead and to the left. The sound of small children chattering away excitedly while they ate their pre dance snacks filled my ears as I walked through the door. I scanned the room and the many lunch tables set up, searching the labels on each table for Nico's teacher's name. In the back of the room, I finally found Nico's homeroom. My eyes resting on my son, sitting at the end of the table with his best friend. He was smiling, quiet, eating his snack, while the other children at the table chattered to each other. Nico watched his classmates, silently enjoying his snack, smiling at them. He was enjoying their conversations, listening to all they had to say.

I walked to the table and wrapped my arms around Nico, kissing him on the cheek. "Hello, my sweet guy," I said to Nico,

39

softly in his ear, just loud enough for him hear me over the chatter filling the cafeteria. "Hi, mom," he replied, eating another Goldfish from his bag of snacks. He took a sip of his water bottle nearby, looked up at me, and smiled, shrugging his shoulders up and down contentedly. Not long after, the lights dimmed, and the children, excited at this cue that the dance was beginning, jumped excitedly out of their seats and made their way to the front of the gym, a large empty area inviting them to dance and begin their hour of fun.

"Come on, Neeks! Let's go dance!" I excitedly said to him. I reached for his hand, and he and I walked together across the floor to the edge of the circle of children, all moving with the beat of the music, smiles on their faces, laughter in the air. I started dancing with Nico. He danced with me, smiling, no words needed. He seemed to be enjoying himself, and I was enjoying my time with him. His eyes sparkled, as they always do. We joined his best friend, who had also found a space to join the circle in the same space where we were. Nico and his friend danced together and laughed. I smiled at Nico. He was having fun.

A few minutes later, a conga line formed among the children, with each child at the dance joining, one at a time. Holding on to the shoulders of the child in front of them, each child joined the conga line as it slowly grew, circling almost entirely around the gym floor. I turned to look at Nico, trying to read whether or not he wanted to join the conga line. He stood back, silent, biting his pinky finger, communicating his nervousness to me. "Come on, Nico," I said to him, as I motioned to the conga line. Trying to encourage him to join, I reached for his hand. He pulled back, showing apprehension, but not altogether disinterested. He stood, instead, silently, watching the conga line of classmates move around him, children laughing and dancing as they moved. He stood and watched. I couldn't help but wonder what he was thinking in this moment. I wanted so badly to tell him how amazing he is. I wanted to tell him that he could do this, that I believed in him. I wondered how hard it must be for him to trust others his age, to try and decide, daily, where he fit into this world, in each situation as it presented himself. I stood and took a deep breath and watched him. I watched him as he waited, I watched him observe. For what seemed like forever, minutes ticked by, the conga line not breaking up, but, instead, growing in size and energy. I reached for his hand once more and smiled at him as his eyes looked deep into mine. "You got this, buddy," I said with my eyes. I gave him a smile, and he looked back at me. Biting his fingers still, he inched forward towards me. Some more time passed, and I didn't break my gaze. He inched forward more, and once again, more, until he was standing next to me. We awaited the end of the conga line, and I, along with Nico, took the shoulders of the last student, and Nico and I moved with the conga line a few steps before moving back out of the line. Nico stepped back away from the line and looked down. I recognized that, at this point, Nico was trying to talk to me, but the music prevented me from hearing him. I leaned forward, gently putting my ear against his mouth so that I could hear him. "I want a drink," he said. "Ok, buddy," I said to him. I reached once more for his hand, and he and I made our way to the cafeteria table where our dance afternoon had begun. I sat down next to him on the cafeteria bench, and he had the rest of his snack and drink, my arm around him. I held him close as he ate. We spent the remainder of our time that afternoon at that table until, a little before the dance was scheduled to end, Nico requested to leave. I took his hand for the last time that afternoon, my heart full of pride and admiration. We made our way to the same cafeteria doors in which I entered early, down the hallway at the entrance of the school, and to the car. It was on this day I learned that courage comes in many ways and under various circumstances, and showing courage is not always easy.

At the dance that afternoon, my son gave me the gift of courage. Courage is found deep within. It is pushing oneself past his comfort zone, growing as he goes. That afternoon, I saw my son try something new, something that made him anxious. He did it. Even for a few minutes, he did it. I can't imagine how much courage it takes to live in this world, a world wired differently than our son understands. To get out of bed each day and tackle this world, school, our community, takes a lot bravery. Nico attending the dance that afternoon and joining that conga line has found a special place my heart. When I am afraid of anything, I think of my son. I think of that dance, of that conga line. If he can do it, I can do it. I can tackle my fears, if even for a few minutes, before deciding whether it is right for me or not. When I doubt myself, or my ability to do something, when I think something is too hard, or not worth the fight, I think of that conga line. My son has inspired and encouraged me, and he's taught me that life is worth fighting for. Situations that force us to grow-they don't come easily. They don't come without bravery, without courage. I could join the conga line and love it, or I could join the conga line and discover that it isn't for me. The only way to do it is to find the shield of armor, the bravery to tackle the scariest things, or things that I find uncomfortable. I carry this gift, this reminder, always with me. I've learned how much I can accomplish from doing things scared. It just took my son and a conga line.

DAYS IN PICTURES

Nico has many amazing qualities. Besides being the kindest, most genuine, brave and hard working person I know, Nico is also a superhero. Not in the pop culture sense, and not in the way you see or hear about in comic books or in movies, with men who can spin webs from their hands, or fly above cities, fighting bad guys and saving the world from evil. No, Nico's superhero abilities come in a different form, in a type of giftedness not uncommon to the world of Autism. Nico is a visual superhero.

On a warm spring day when Nico was six years old, we took a trip to Nico's grandmother's house, about a 45-minute drive away. The sky that day was a brilliant blue, and spring was in full bloom. Flowers and leaves were budding from the trees, the warm spring air filled with the scent of pollen and the promise of summer, situated just around the corner. We were equipped with sunscreen and light spring clothes, as it was sure that the plans for the day would certainly include time outside in Nicos' grandmother's backyard. What better way to spend a spring day than playing on the swings, enjoying some barbecued foods, followed by watermelon and fresh fruit for dessert. The day set before us was sure to be an enjoyable one.

We exited the car at my mother-in-law's house, and as I started towards the backyard, I realized Nico was still standing next to the van, his eyes fixed on the trees lining the back of the yard. His head was tilted so that his eyes gazed at the tops of the trees, as if he was almost working out the details of something small in the trees. He was entranced by whatever it was he saw, and I, now, also joined him in his observing. I wonder what he was looking at, I thought to myself. "Nico, do you see the trees?" His eyes remained stuck on the treetops as he said to me, in a soft voice, "The circle in the trees." "The circle in the trees?" I repeated, both puzzled. I looked closer and turned again to see the direction in which his gaze was pointed. The circle in the trees, I thought. Well, a lot of things in a tree are circular in shape. I wondered if maybe he saw a bird's nest, or a knot in the wood. I looked back at the trees, squinting in the hopes of getting a better idea of what was catching his attention so intensely. "Maybe it is a bird's nest," I said to him. "A circle in the tree," he repeated. I, once again, looked at the trees, but couldn't see a circle in the tree. Figuring he must see a shape of a branch somewhere, or, maybe a bird's nest that I couldn't find, I figured it was better to validate what he saw than to question it. It was important to him, after all, and therefore, it was important to me. "Yes, a circle in the tree." I said to him. "Come on. Let's go see Grandma." I took his hand

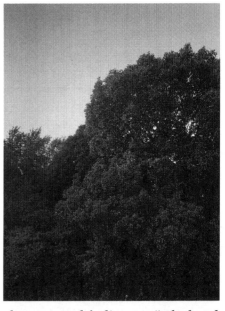

and let him to the backyard, noticing that, for the entire walk, he continued to look at the treetops, at the exact spot on which his eyes fixed when he stood beside the van. He saw something. Something special had caught his eye. I wondered what it was.

For the remainder of that afternoon, Nico continued to look up at the trees. He told each member of our family about the "circle in the tree." HIs grandparents, his uncles, his aunts, they all looked at the tree tops. "I think he is referring to the branch shapes or a bird's nest," I helped to clarify. "Whatever it is, it must be interesting. He really seems to enjoy it." Our family members would take this explanation as satisfactory, and would either give Nico a kiss or knowing smile, each member of our family, a strong support system in our son's life and in ours. For hours, Nico continued to be mesmerized by the "circle in the tree." As the evening wore on, Nico watched the "circle in the tree." He noted it, time and time again. Day turned to evening, and as the evening went on, and darkness took over the blue sky, transforming it to a dark blue and eventual black, Nico's interest in the tree tops subsided. Before long, it was time to head home. We all said goodbye to our family, our day together coming to an end. My fascination with what Nico saw that day, however, did not.

The next few weeks, whenever we were outside, and trees were nearby, Nico would talk about the "circle in the tree." He would peer at the treetops and point, announcing what he saw. My suspicion that the "circle" was a bird's nest or a specific knot in the wood in one of the trees in my mother-in-law's backyard had now faded, as he noticed this "circle" in multiple tree species, with multiple branch shapes, and in none of the trees could I ever find a nest. My curiosity grew along with Nico's findings. At the park, in our backyard, at a friend's house, Nico noticed and identified the "circle in the tree." It was a few weeks later, when it finally clicked. The "circle in the tree"-it was the circle made by the branch, or branches, with the sky behind it. It was, indeed, a circle. In the tree. In other words, he noticed the circles made when branches don't quite meet each other. He noticed the way the sky peeked through the branches, pieces of parts of clouds being visible, and the blue sky making an appearance in between groups of leaves. You may have seen this same shape in a tree when the tree has lost most of its branches, wrapping around the light source behind it. Instead of seeing the tree as branches with the sky in the background, our son saw it as a number of circles, both green and blue, depending on where the sky appeared. It occurred to me, at this point, that our son was visually gifted, a conclusion proven true time and time again since then, when he shows us he can remember the spelling of very large, complicated words after seeing them just once, or the way he remembers numbers on hotel room doors, or how he sees shapes and objects in otherwise normal, everyday store logos. He sees animals in the shape of a logo of a nearby shoe store, or a fish in the outline of a gymnast at my daughter's gym. He sees an entirely new world in things the rest of us skip over.

Nico has given me the gift of being able to see things in a different way. He has taught me that there is more than meets the eye. Everyday situations, things that become commonplace to us, they are comprised of another layer. There is more than one way to look our whole world, our day-to-day interactions with others, and even our circumstances. Whenever I'm faced with what seems like a one-sided situation, I stop. I pause, even for just a second. And I've learned to look for the "circle in the tree." The alternate view, even the message that lies within. I try to approach situations with an open mind, knowing that to some, an outline of a gymnast can look like both a girl standing on her toes, and, to others, maybe a fish, with its tail down and its mouth in the air. Nico has taught me that this entire world, and all situations we face, there are two or more sides to every story. Sometimes, things we seek to understand, or answers to problems we face, are in plain sight. They are right before us, hidden in a layer we were not able to see before. I never knew how to pay close enough attention to the branches of the trees to see how the sky peeked through the branches. To me, they were just green with sky behind them. Now, I see trees as holes, or shapes, of green and blue, and even sometimes white. Because of Nico, I am lucky enough to see trees in a way most do not. Trees, and the sky, in shapes, and the rest of the world from more than one angle. Thank you, Nico.

A BLANKET FORT

It was a lazy Saturday morning, the kind where the soft hum of television shows make part of the soundtrack, the smell of coffee filling the air, the quietness following a hectic week, a perfect springboard into a few days at home before the week ahead of us picked up. There wasn't much to do to start our weekend, and we all had somehow crawled out of our beds and made it to the same destination-the couch, with blankets and throw pillows, all six of us cozying in together, finding comfort in some relaxation time as a family.

After some time, the children, having had their fill of cuddling, left the room, moving instead to the toy room. One by one, they left the comfort of the couch in search of toys with which to play, books to read, or pages to color. Our Saturday morning movie ending, I finally stood up from the couch to go and start some laundry, when I realized that the blankets, all strewn about the couch only an hour or so before, were missing. Intending on including them in my Saturday morning load of laundry, I looked, at first, around the family room, assuming they had fallen either behind the couch or were thrown to the side, hiding between the couch and wall. My search proved fruitless, as I couldn't find a single blanket that had been there just this morning. I looked up, and, simultaneously, heard laughing coming from the toy room. I walked over and looked around the corner. Ahh, the blankets. Tied up to each corner of the couch, propped up on the toy shelves with heavy toys, laid delicately on the top of larger toys. A blanket fort. This particular blanket fort was not like any other I had seen. It was large, complex, and, from the looks of it, delicate, yet strong. It was obvious that the children built this fort with great care. I peeked inside as our third-born popped up. He took me on a "tour" of the interior. They had built rooms inside, dragging play food into to make a kitchen, and their own shoes lined one wall in order to mark the entry. They had included some smaller toys in one corner of the fort to indicate that this is where the toy room was, and they even included some artwork they had made earlier in the week. Coloring book pages, one from each child, lay spread out, propped up against one wall of the fort. I smiled. I was amazed at their creativity, and the size and scope of this blanket fort instantly transferred me to days of my childhood, where it became a mission, a task, to build a blanket fort like none other. I dropped to my knees and pushed the edge of one blanket, a corner that had been hanging in front of my face, to the side. All four of my children were lying on their stomachs, side by side, laughing at pictures and videos they were taking of themselves on the ipad. They were huddled together, arms around each other's shoulders, some of them making "peace signs" at the camera as it snapped. Their giggles made my heart soar. I loved the way that they all played together. I loved so much the way that Nico had a place he belonged, his siblings always protecting him, carefully, delicately, much in the same way the blanket fort was constructed. They covered him, protected him, and made him feel safe. Another snapshot with the iPad, and more giggles. They were laughing with each other, enjoying each other's company. Nico, thrown right into the mix. This place in his life, a constant, steady source of safety. Nico's siblings are his champions, and he, theirs.

Nico's three siblings play an integral part in his life, providing for him many gifts. They are the ones that show him what true friendship feels like, and they are the first ones to see him and know him for all of the amazing things he is. They cheer him on, in both official and unofficial ways. They are in the stands at his hockey games, they congratulate him when he wins a game of war. They lead him. They show him how to do things, like play video games, and they help him cut cookies into heart and star shapes with the cookie cutter. They show him what kindness looks and feels like. They hug him every morning, and hide under blanket forts with him, snapping

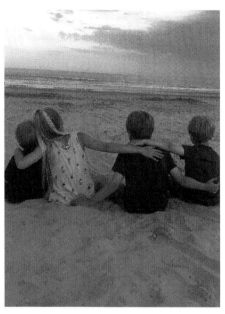

pictures with the iPad, enjoying time as friends. They include him in their games, they ask him how he feels, they pay attention to him and respect him. They show him all of the goodness this world has to offer, each and every day. They protect him. On the bus each morning, they sit with him, even when their other friends request that they sit somewhere else. They take him by the hand to accompany him on the slide at the playground, and they stick by him. If he wants to play inside, they stay with him. They make it so he isn't alone. He doesn't need to leave or look anywhere for his best friends. They are with him always. They've taught him what goodness in others looks like, and they are his safe zone. They are his tribe.

Nico also learns some of the tough lessons of life, too. He learns about sharing, about how to deal with jealousy, and he learns about the law of natural consequences when he fights with them or takes toys, as most children do. He's learned strategies from them, coping mechanisms to deal with some of the more complicated aspects of life. He's learned how to compromise, how to work through frustration when people with whom you are close to disagree. He's developed an understanding of how to get along with others.

Nico, too, plays an integral part in their lives, and the gifts he offers them are many. Nico has taught them to see the world in a different way. My children have developed hearts and minds that are open, knowing that it is the many different approaches to life and to living that make this world so special. They've grown up knowing that not everyone is the same, and, more importantly, they've learned how truly great this is. They are learning to lead and see the world with their hearts. They've been given some amazing and unique experiences, too, all because of their brother. Attending professional hockey games, riding on parade floats, participating in dog training sessions, and meeting some of the coolest people on Earth highlight the list. Growing up with Nico has made my children infinitely better people. They will go into this world someday having learned lessons some people never learn in a lifetime. They will be equipped to make this world a better place, all because of Nico. In this blanket fort, on this slow, Saturday morning, I saw a complicated, intricate love. A love, like the blanket fort, that protects, that takes care and delicate hands and hearts to foster. The love between siblings.

A BOW ON THE TOP

To my son, I owe my most sincere gratitude. His very existence is a source of inspiration for many, a constant ray of sunshine in my life and his family's life, and a reminder that beautiful things await those who simply open their eyes, taking in all life has to offer. As a conclusion to this book, as a culminating bow on the collection of gifts given to us by him, I write Nico this thank you letter.

To my dear son...

Thank you for all of the gifts you give us daily, the gifts that come from you being exactly who you are. Much like the kite you were flying on the beach one day, may you continue to fly high, dipping and soaring with the direction of the winds. I hope your colors, bright and true, continue to catch people's eyes, grabbing their attention, and filling them with hope. Your ability to bend and flow with the winds teaches us all how to use courage to achieve our dreams. The tattered strings on your tail make up a small but notable part of you, making you unique and allowing you to catch the winds in a different way than other kites do, but they don't stop you from achieving great things, performing great tricks in the air. For now, we all all stand and watch, learning from you as you fly high, as you soar to the clouds and beyond. Thank you, Nico.

Love,

Mommy

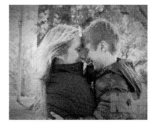

GIFTS ARE SPECIAL

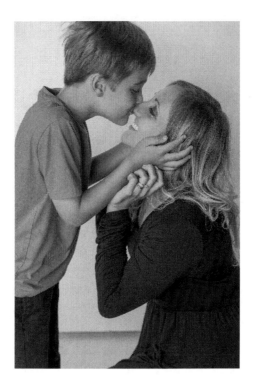

They are often unexpected, and they bring us great joy.
May you find the gifts in everyday life like I have.

ABOUT THE AUTHOR

Dana Bauer

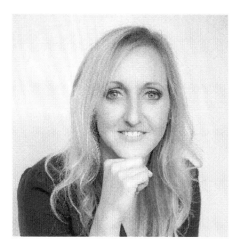

Dana is a parent dedicated to making this world a better place for her son and millions of others with Autism Spectrum Disorder. She resides in Pittsburgh, Pennsylvania with her husband and four children. Visit her website at www.navigating-nico.com for more resources and inspriation.

Made in the USA
Columbia, SC
09 November 2020

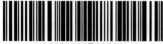